Book 1:

The Hyperthyroidism Handbook

BY LINDSEY P

&

Book 2:

The Hypothyroidism Handbook

BY LINDSEY P

Book 1:

The Hyperthyroidism Handbook

BY LINDSEY P

An Everyday Guide to Natural Solutions of Living with Hyperthyroidism including Weight Gain, Increased Energy and General Well-being

THE
HYPERTHYROIDISM
HANDBOOK

An everyday guide to natural solutions of living with hyperthyroidism, including weight gain, increased energy and general well-being

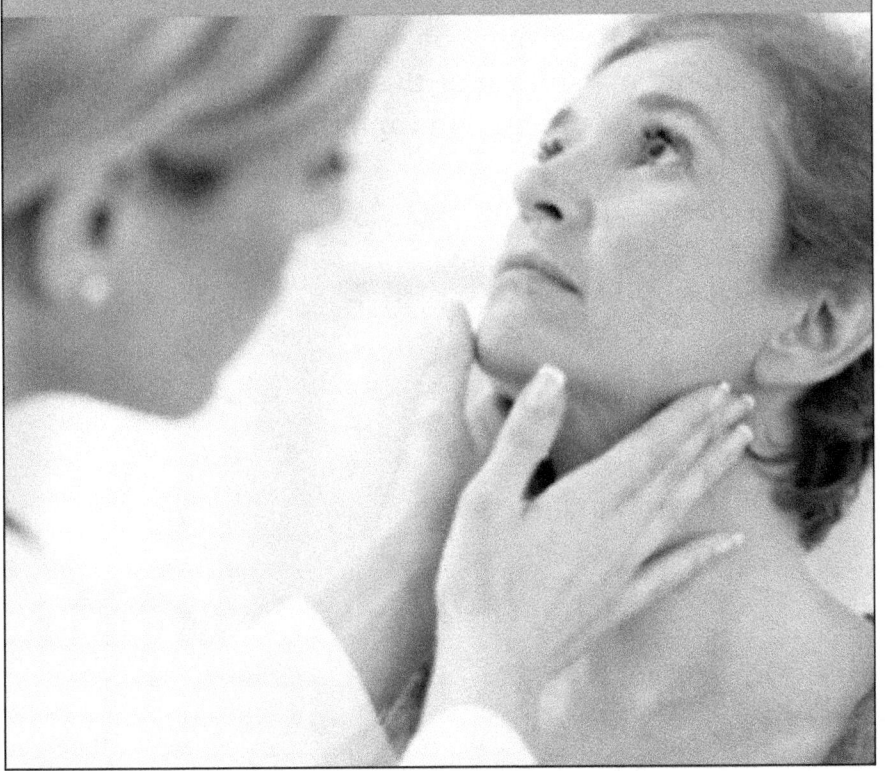

Table of Contents

Introduction

I want to thank you and congratulate you for purchasing the book, *"The Hyperthyroidism Handbook: An Everyday Guide to Natural Solutions of Living with Hyperthyroidism including Weight Gain, Increased Energy and General Well-being"*.

This book contains proven steps and strategies on how to recognize and diagnose hyperthyroidism based on the signs and symptoms at an early stage to prevent the worsening of the disorder. If in case the disorder has progressed already, this book serves as an ultimate guide on how to live with hyperthyroidism in the best and healthiest possible ways.

Hyperthyroidism is a disease of the thyroid gland. This book is not intended as a medical substitute. It only serves as a guide on how life can be easier for someone who suffers from the disease. Medical help is very important and patients should first seek medical attention.

Comprehensive information on hyperthyroidism is provided on this book. Readers will know how hyperthyroidism is diagnosed, treated and what causes it. Knowledge of the disease should not be limited to doctors alone. It is especially important for the patient and his family members to be knowledgeable about the disease so that they can help the patient avoid the things that should be avoided and pursue all the things that can lead to the betterment of the patient's general health and well-being.

Thanks again for purchasing this book, I hope you enjoy it!

Chapter 1: Hyperthyroidism Defined

Overactive thyroid is also another popular name for hyperthyroidism. This condition is characterized by the excessive production and secretion of the thyroid hormones known as T3 or triiodothyronine and T4 or thyroxine – free hormones secreted by the thyroid gland which are not protein-bound and are released into the blood stream. The most popular cause of this condition is the Grave's disease (which will be further discussed on the causes of hyperthyroidism) and the opposite condition is called the sluggish thyroid otherwise known as the hypothyroidism for it is characterized by a reduction in the production and secretion of the thyroid hormones T3 and T4.

An overactive thyroid is the result of a clinical syndrome known as thyrotoxicosis that occurs when the serum levels of T3 and T4 are unusually high in the bloodstream. Thyrotoxicosis however, can still develop in the absence of hyperthyroidism. When there is an inflamed thyroid gland- a condition known as thyroiditis- thyrotoxicosis occurs as the stored hormones in the swollen thyroid gland are released in excessive amounts even without the production of T3 and T4 which characterizes hyperthyroidism. Furthermore, the condition thyrotoxicosis can develop as a result of too much ingestion of the levothyroxine which is an exogenous thyroid hormone sold in the market as a supplementary thyroid hormone. This phenomenon is clinically dubbed as alimentary thyrotoxicosis, exogenous thyrotoxicosis or occult factitial thyrotoxicosis.

Although hyperthyroidism causes thyrotoxicosis, the therapy and treatment as well as the medical management of the disease is different from the thyrotoxicosis caused by other condition and that which is caused by hyperthyroidism. Different methods are utilized clinically to diagnose and apply appropriate treatments such as radiotracer thyroid measurements and thyroid imaging.

Thyroid Hormones and the Process:

Cell metabolism is stimulated by the thyroid hormones which are produced by the thyroid gland. The thyroid gland is situated below the adam's apple in men and at the lower part of the neck in women and children just above the collar bones. It is shaped like a butterfly complete with the two lobes that form like wings and the isthmus which looks like the body of the butterfly. The thyroid gland envelops the trachea or the wind pipe.

The thyroid gland functions by extracting iodine in the blood which then uses it in the production of the thyroid hormones. Iodine is the primary component needed by the thyroid gland to function normally. It comes from the food we eat like salt, bread and seafood. The 2 most important hormones produced by the thyroid gland are triiodothyronine or T3 and the thyroxine or the T4. 99.9 percent of the hormones produced by the thyroid gland consist of the T4 while .1 percent is T3. Although T3 constitute only .01 % of the hormones produced by the thyroid gland, it is the most active or potent hormone as it has the biggest impact on the body. It has the most biological activity when released in the bloodstream. Since it is more important than the T4, most T4 hormones will then be converted to T-3 when it reaches the bloodstream to complement the necessity for active hormones in the body.

The Process:

There is a chain of command being followed in the regulation of thyroid hormones. It is not surprising because the human body is governed by different internal processes. The thyroid gland is regulated by the pituitary gland, which is another gland located in the brain. Similarly, the pituitary gland is regulated by the thyroid gland in a 'feedback' effect of thyroid hormones in the pituitary. Both glands are then regulated by the hypothalamus, which is another important gland located in the brain.

The hypothalamus releases thyrotropin (TRH) which signals the pituitary gland to release the thyroid-stimulating hormones (TSH). Once TSH is released in the bloodstream, the thyroid gland will then release thyroid hormones which are T3 and T4. If there are any disruptions the supply of the hormones will be reduced causing hypothyroidism. But if there is another condition, like grave's disease, the thyroid gland will release excessive amounts of T3 and T4 resulting to hyperthyroidism.

The pituitary gland controls thyroid hormone production. As a result, if there's insufficient supply of thyroid hormone circulating in the blood stream for normal cell metabolism, the pituitary gland will attempt to balance the insufficiency by producing more thyroid-stimulating hormones (TSH) to stimulate more thyroid hormone production. In contrast, if there's excessive amount of thyroid hormones in the blood, the pituitary gland will decrease the production of TSH to lower the production of thyroid hormones.

Chapter 2: What are the Causes of Hyperthyroidism?

Several factors can cause hyperthyroidism. Oftentimes, when the entire thyroid gland malfunctions it results to the overproduction of thyroid hormones. Excessive secretion of the thyroid hormones may also be a result of a single 'hot' nodule. Thyroiditis which is an inflammation of the thyroid also causes hyperthyroidism. Aside from these causes, there are other clinical conditions that may result to hyperthyroidism. These are the following:

1. **Grave's Disease**: It is an autoimmune disease which may be characterized by different levels of iodine found in the human diet. This phenomenon results to the thyroid's over-activity which then causes hyperthyroidism. A person diagnosed with Grave's disease has a thyroid gland which cannot respond properly to the command or signals sent by the pituitary glands through the secretion of the Thyroid stimulating hormones or TSH. Women are five times more susceptible to this disease than men. It is also hereditary. Diagnosis includes the detection of antibodies like TSI or thyroid stimulating immunoglobulin, TSH receptor antibodies and the thyroid peroxidase antibodies which are believed to be inherent to the disease.

   Grave's disease can be triggered by many factors. These include: radiation to the neck, stress, medications, smoking and viral infections. Standard diagnosis makes use of the nuclear medicine known as thyroid scan/imaging. This method can capture images of the increased levels of the iodine in the blood which are initially labeled with radioactive sensors. Blood test is also used to determine the elevated levels of TSI in the blood.

Aside from hyperthyroidism, Grave's disease can also cause skin lesions or dermopathy and eye disease known as Grave's ophthalmopathy which can occur on, before or after hyperthyroidism is diagnosed. Ophthalmopathy is characterized by a feeling of sand in the eyes, double vision, sensitivity to light, and protruded eyes. Those who smoke generally experience worse symptoms. In treating ophthalmopathy, surgery may be required as well as steroid therapy to regulate the inflammation. Lastly, dermopathy is quite rare and when it does occur, it is usually painless. The rash is reddish and lumpy and it usually occurs on the frontal area of the legs.

2. **Toxic multinodular goiter and adenoma**: As people age, the thyroid gland becomes naturally lumpy. These lumps are natural and they require no medical attention as they do not produce any thyroid hormones. There are times when a nodule starts to grow bigger than the rest (more than 3cm) and may become autonomous in the process. When a nodule becomes autonomous, it produces hormones independently and does not respond to the signals from the pituitary gland through the thyroid stimulating hormones (TSH). This single nodule may not have any serious impact on the thyroid but when more than one nodule becomes larger and autonomous, the phenomenon becomes toxic and

these functioning nodules are detected by a thyroid scanner.

3. **Thyroiditis**: This is known as the inflammation of the thyroid. There are 2 most popular type of Thyroiditis. One is the Hashimoto's Thyroiditis which is a common condition leading to hypothyroidism and the Subacute Thyroiditis which generally occurs after a viral infection. Subacute Thyroiditis is characterized by a sore throat and painful swallowing coupled with a fever. When touched, the thyroid is tender. Neck pains may be reported as well. Another type of Thyroiditis may develop known as the lymphocytic Thyroiditis where lymphocytes or white blood cells may accumulate in the inflamed gland. When this happens, the thyroid gland becomes 'leaky' resulting to an increased level of hormones in the blood. Lymphocytic Thyroiditis commonly develops after pregnancy and 8 percent after delivery. After delivery, the hyperthyroid stage usually lasts up to 12 weeks and will then be succeeded by hypothyroid phase which lasts up to 6 months. After this phase, the woman goes back to normal thyroid functioning.

4. **Thyroid Hormones excessive intake:** Patients who are taking some oral thyroid hormones usually take in larger doses because their medications are not properly monitored. Some patients fail to make a follow-up with their doctors so they tend to consume excess thyroid hormones as indicated. There are also instances where the patient overindulge and abuse the medication for weight loss purposes.

5. **Intake of Amiodarone:** This drug is quite similar to thyroxin and intake can result to over or under activity of the thyroid.

6. **Postpartum Thyroiditis**: This occurs in women and affects 7% of those who gave birth. PPT starts with the hyperthyroidism phase which lasts up to a few weeks to a few months and then goes back to normal.

7. **Struma Ovarii**: Monodermal teratoma which is rarely detected and contains mostly thyroid tissue that results to hyperthyroidism.

8. **Iodine excessive consumption**: This may be a result of over-eating of foods rich in iodine such as kelp, salt, and other seafood. Similarly, a drug known as amiodarone contain iodine and intake of such can increase the level of iodine in the blood.

9. **Over-secretion of the TSH in the blood**: At least 1 percent of hyperthyroidism cases is caused by an abnormal secretion of the thyroid-stimulating hormone in the blood by the pituitary gland. This happens when there is a tumor in the pituitary gland. More TSH in the blood signals the thyroid gland to release more thyroid hormones that leads to hyperthyroidism. This phenomenon may also be associated with other conditions associated with the pituitary and an endocrinologist typically performs a series of tests to detect the problem.

Chapter 3: Signs and Symptoms of Hyperthyroidism

Medically speaking hyperthyroidism is characterized by excessive thyroid hormones in the bloodstream. Physiologically, thyroid hormones play a very important role in the metabolic processes that govern the cellular functions. They affect nearly all types of body tissues. They serve to control the physiological processes in the body otherwise known as the metabolic rate.

Consequently, the amount of thyroid hormones dictates the pace of these metabolic processes. The more thyroid hormones in the blood the faster the processes can become. This is precisely the reason why patients who have hyperthyroidism experience the symptoms of: irritability, nervousness, increased heart rate, increased perspiration, anxiety, sleeping difficulties, hand tremors, fine and brittle hair, skin-thinning and muscular weaknesses in the areas of the thigh and upper arms. Diarrhea is reported to be uncommon but frequent bowel movement is more likely. Despite good appetite, considerable weight loss is detected although 10% are more likely to gain weight. Vomiting also is included and women may experience abnormalities in their menstrual flow such as period becoming less frequent or flows may be less heavy.

Increased levels of thyroid hormones in the blood also cause palpitations and increased heart rate similar to that of epinephrine overdose. Other symptoms include: anxiety, hand tremors, hyper-motility of the digestive system, low serum cholesterol and unintended weight loss.

Most common clinical signs and symptoms include: weight loss despite good appetite, hair loss (outer third of the eyebrows), intolerance to heat, fatigue, weakness, muscle aches, hyperglycemia, irritability, hyperactivity, delirium, myxedema (in case of Grave's disease), polyuria, pretibial and sweating. Others include: difficulty to concentrate, panic attacks and memory problems.

In case of a thyroid storm, the patient experiences paranoia and psychosis but these are less common in cases of hyperthyroidism. Complete reduction of the symptoms is commonly experienced by many during 1-2 months after the period of euthyroid is obtained. Physical symptoms include: shortness of breath, loss of libido, palpitations, vomiting, nausea, feminization and diarrhea. If untreated for long-term, hyperthyroidism may lead to osteoporosis.

There were also a number of neurological signs and symptoms established. These include: periodic paralysis (more common in people with Asian descent), tremors, myopathy and chorea. Myasthenia Gravis and hyperthyroidism has also been found to be quite connected. 5% of myasthenic patients have hyperthyroidism. Even after thyroid treatment, myasthenia cannot be cured because it is auto-immune.

As the most common cause of hyperthyroidism, Grave's disease presents other underlying symptoms. This includes the enlargement of the eyes due to the swelling of eye muscles. This symptom can only be treated with surgical procedures. Both eyes may be protruded and some patients have goiter due to enlarged thyroid gland.

Other minor ocular symptoms of hyperthyroidism include: lid-lag, eyelid retraction and extra-ocular muscle weakness.

Dalrymple sign or hyperthyroid stare, the eyelids are abnormally retracted upward. Extra-ocular muscle weakness results to double vision. In patients with lid-lag symptoms, the eyelids fail to follow the directions taken by the iris especially when the iris goes downward following a moving object. This is temporary though, and will eventually disappear after treatment.

Lastly, Grave's disease comes with exophthalmos or protrusion of the eyelids. Exophthalmos occurs exclusively to hyperthyroidism caused by Grave's disease although not all exophthalmic symptoms are diagnostic of Grave's disease. With hyperthyroidism, the immune-mediated swelling of the retro-orbital socket (eye socket) causes the eyes to protrude.

Chapter 4: How is Hyperthyroidism Diagnosed?

When hyperthyroidism is suspected, the initial test will be the measurement of the TSH (thyroid-stimulating hormones) in the blood. If the TSH level is low, this is an indication that the pituitary gland is signaled by the brain (hypothalamus) to reduce the secretion of the hormones as it detected an increased level of T3 and T4 in the blood. In other occasions, low levels of TSH in the blood are indicative of pituitary malfunction or temporary reticence of the pituitary gland due to other medical conditions. This is why TSH measurement is the most important first step to consider.

Diagnosis may also be contributed by the measurement of antibodies associated with the thyroid gland such as anti-TSH receptor antibodies (commonly found in Grave's disease) and the anti-thyroid peroxidase (indicative of Hashimoto's Thyroiditis).

Such diagnosis will only be confirmed when the blood test shows that there is indeed an increased level of T3 and T4 in the blood as well as the reduced level of TSH in the blood. The pituitary gland regulates the amount of thyroid hormones released by the thyroid gland. If there's too much thyroid hormone, the pituitary gland will reduce the level of TSH in the blood instructing the thyroid gland to reduce the thyroid hormones production. The cause of hyperthyroidism can be diagnosed using the thyroid scan as well as the radioactive iodine uptake. The uptake test utilizes radioactive iodine which may be taken orally or injected on an empty stomach to come up with the measurement of iodine being absorbed by the thyroid gland. If the iodine absorption is too much, this means the person has hyperthyroidism. Thyroid scans allow the radiologists and endocrinologists to have a visual examination of the overactive thyroid.

To differentiate hyperthyroidism from Thyroiditis, a method known as scintigraphy is used. There will be two tests connected to each other including the uptake test and the thyroid imaging with the use of gamma camera. Uptake test, as mentioned before uses radioactive iodine (iodine-123 is the most commonly preferred radionuclide but iodine-131 is the traditional radionuclide being used). Iodine-123 is the perfect isotope of iodine for the thyroid tissue imaging and thyroid cancer metastasis.

The administration of this radioactive iodine involves oral consumption of a pill or liquid which contains sodium iodide (NaI) consisting of a small amount of iodine-123. The patient is required to fast for 2 hours prior and 1 hour after the pill ingestion. This method is safe unless the patient has allergic reactions to iodine. The excess radioiodine which was not absorbed by the thyroid gland will then be excreted from the body through urinating. If an allergic reaction occurs, the patient will be given an antihistamine.

After 24 hours, the patient is expected to return for the uptake test. This method utilizes a device with a metal bar placed against the neck that can measure the emitted radioactivity by the thyroid gland. The test takes only 4 minutes until the percentage of the uptake is accumulated and measured by the software. Simultaneous scanning is also taking place where imaging is derived including the left, right and central angle with a gamma camera. The radiologists will be the one to read and interpret the imaging and the report will be filed including the uptake examination results and comments about the imaging. Radioactive iodine intake is usually higher in patients with hyperthyroidism.

Lastly, other doctors test the T3, free T3, T4 and/or Free T4 to come up with better and more accurate results. If the T3 and T4 levels are higher than normal in the blood that indicates that the person has hyperthyroidism.

Chapter 5: How is Hyperthyroidism Treated?

Hyperthyroidism cases typically require an initial treatment using the anti-thyroid drugs or medically known as the suppressive thyrostatics medication. Use of anti-thyroid drugs is temporary. At a more advanced stage, however, radioisotope therapy or surgical procedure may be conducted to permanently resolve hyperthyroidism issues. Unfortunately, all these treatments may cause the thyroid gland to become underactive leading to the opposite condition known as hypothyroidism. When that happens, triiodothyronine and levothyroxine may be taken as supplements to manage the side effects. Surgical options are necessary especially when the thyroid gland is enlarged and may be posing some threats to underlying tissues due to the neck compression structures or when hyperthyroidism is triggered as an effect of a more cancerous origin.

Here are the treatments used to combat hyperthyroidism:

1. **Anti-thyroid drugs**: These are drugs that are powerful enough to reduce the production of thyroid hormones. Examples of these drugs are: propylthiouracil, methimazole (sold in the US) and carbimazole (sold in the UK). These anti-thyroid drugs work by slowing down the iodination of thyroglobulin and in effect will reduce the production of T4 or tetraiodothyronine. Propylthiouracil, on the other hand, prevents the conversion of T4 to T3 outside the thyroid gland when it reaches the bloodstream. It is important to note though, anti-thyroid drugs take effect after a few weeks because of

the substantial amount of thyroid hormone stored in the thyroid tissue. The dosage need to be carefully monitored for a period of one month coupled with doctor follow-up and blood tests.

Initially, a high dose is recommended but if it persisted, hypothyroidism may develop as a result. Block and replace method is also administered to patients where they will be given sufficient dosage of anti-thyroid drugs to block the hormone production completely and then the patients will be treated as hypothyroidism patients.

2. **Food and Diet**: Hyperthyroidism patients cannot be given foods rich I iodine such as kelps and seaweeds. Iodized salts are also believed to have no desired effect but instead it has increased the number of deaths in the United States so that has to be eliminated in the case of hyperthyroidism patients.

3. **Beta-Blockers**: Since hyperthyroidism affects nearly all processes in the body and resulting oftentimes to increased heart rate, palpitations, sweating and the likes, beta-blockers are recommended to tame these symptoms and help the patient to calm down. They regulate the heart beat and minimize the onset of palpitations, hand tremors and anxiety. Beta-blockers offer temporary relief from these symptoms until the procedure of the radioiodine is administered. They do not treat and therefore cannot be used to treat hyperthyroidism. They can only reduce the symptoms.

Propranolol can also be used to minimize the onset of symptoms. L-propranolol treats the symptoms associated with the nerves such as tremors, anxiety, palpitations and heat intolerance. D-propranolol, on the other hand, blocks the conversion of T4 to T3. Propanolol is most commonly used in the UK while metoprolol is used in the US but both are helpful in treating hyperthyroid patients' symptoms.

4. **Surgery**: Thyroidectomy is a surgical procedure that refers to removing the thyroid gland whether the entire gland or just a part of it. Surgery is the last method used when all else failed but most often, cases are treated and resolved by just administering the radioactive iodine method. Surgical procedures are more complicated because it involves the removal of the parathyroid glands and cutting of the laryngeal nerve resulting to a difficulty in swallowing. There may also be an increased risk of acquiring staphylococcal infection as with any major surgeries. In case of Grave's disease where patients are unable to tolerate the medication and/or allergic to medication especially the radioiodine, surgical procedures are obtained.

5. **Radioiodine**: This is also known as iodine-131 isotope therapy pioneered by Dr. Saul Hertz where the patient is given the radioactive iodine in the form of a pill or liquid which they will have to take in orally. Such method is used once to severely disrupt or completely ruin the function of a hyperactive thyroid gland. Iodine-131 is potentially more potent than iodine-123 (which has a biological half-life from 8-13 hours) for it has a biological half life of up to 8 days. Iodine-131 emits beta particles which are more extremely damaging to the tissues at short range. Once the radioiodine or iodine-131 is administered,

the cells will absorb it resulting to their destruction which will eventually render the thyroid gland mostly if not completely inactive.

There are no side effects to this kind of therapy as the destruction is local. Iodine is easily absorbed by the thyroid cells especially the cells of the hyperactive thyroid. It has been constantly used for 50 years since it has started and the only restrictions include pregnancy and breastfeeding as the breast tissues also pick up iodine). After radioiodine therapy, the patient will then be given the supplemental thyroid hormones to complement the body's requirement. A medical report suggests however, that there's a bigger risk of cancer incidents in patients after the radioiodine therapy.

Radioiodine treatment has a bigger chance of success than ordinary medications. The success rate differs and is dependent on the dosage administered and the cause of hyperthyroidism but generally the success rate is between 75-100 percent. In patients suffering from Grave's disease, the major side-effect of the radioiodine treatment is the occurrence of the life-long hypothyroidism which requires a daily treatment or intake of thyroid hormone. Those with eye disease also experience worsening of the condition after the radioiodine treatment. This is one of the reasons why some patients prefer to have the surgical treatment. In other situations where the patient has a different type of disease, or a larger thyroid gland, or if the first treatment did not take effect, the patient may be given another radioactive treatment. It is not surprising to know that many patients feel unhappy about the idea of taking thyroid hormones for the rest of their lives. Even so, thyroid hormones are generally safe, easy to consume, inexpensive, and very much similar to the thyroid hormone created by the thyroid.

It is quite normal for patients who have undergone radioiodine treatment to experience a worsening effect of the hyperthyroidism symptoms for a few weeks to a few months. This is the result of the total destruction of the thyroid tissue where thyroid hormones are released into the blood as thyroid cells containing these hormones are destroyed as well. If this happens, beta-blockers can definitely reduce the symptoms and make it more tolerable for a period of time.

Majority of the patients do not however, encounter any other problems. Some only complain of a little soreness in the throat area or tenderness of the neck but after a few days it will just disappear without any other associated symptoms.

In case of lactating mothers, it is not advised for them to continue breastfeeding for at least a week as radioiodine may still be present in the milk even after the radioiodine treatment.

78 percent of people treated with radioiodine that has Grave's disease develop hypothyroidism and 40 percent of those who have goiter or toxic multinodular goiter and adenoma swing to sluggish thyroid gland condition. To reduce the rate of failure, it is recommended that dosage should be increased for a more potent effect.

Chapter 6: Thyroid Storm and Hypothyroidism

Other conditions that may have any significant connection with hyperthyroidism are thyroid storm and hypothyroidism. Thyroid storm is a condition where hyperthyroidism symptoms occur at the extremes. Aggressive treatment of resuscitation including a combination of the treatments mentioned above plus an intravenous administration of beta-blockers (such as propranolol, succeeded by thioamide (methimazole)) and an iodine solution or iodinated radio contrast agent plus a steroid known as hydrocortisone is administered intravenously.

Thyroid storm is a severe form of hyperthyroidism associated with irregular heartbeats, diarrhea, vomiting, high temperature and mental agitation. It is a medical emergency where hospital treatments and care facilities are required as it is potentially fatal.

Hypothyroidism, on the other hand is the opposite condition of hyperthyroidism. It is connected to hyperthyroidism because most often, people who have been treated with radioiodine develop hypothyroidism as a side effect to the treatment. It is quite expected as the thyroid gland is damaged. Hypothyroidism case is not at all difficult to manage. A regular intake of thyroid hormone is enough to treat this condition.

Conclusion

Thank you again for purchasing this book!

I hope this book was able to help you to differentiate the different medical conditions which may have some sort of connection to hyperthyroidism. I hope that by reading this eBook, you will be better off equipped with medical knowledge that you can impart or share with those you love who apparently are suffering the same fate.

Your new-found learning about hyperthyroidism will greatly help you in overcoming the negative effects of this condition and you can certainly help out in making sure that medications are properly administered to the patient.

The next step is to share this information with the people you love. You can also inspire others to read this eBook so that they, too can learn what you have learned.

Finally, if you enjoyed this book, please take the time to share your thoughts and post a review on Amazon. We do our best to reach out to readers and provide the best value we can. Your positive review will help us achieve that. It'd be greatly appreciated!

Thank you and good luck!

Book 2:

The Hypothyroidism Handbook:

BY LINDSEY P

An Everyday Guide to Natural Solutions of living with Hypothyroidism including increased energy, lasting weight loss, and general well-being

THE
HYPOTHYROIDISM
HANDBOOK

An everyday guide to natural solutions of living with

Hypothyroidism including Increased Energy, lasting

Weight Loss and general well-being

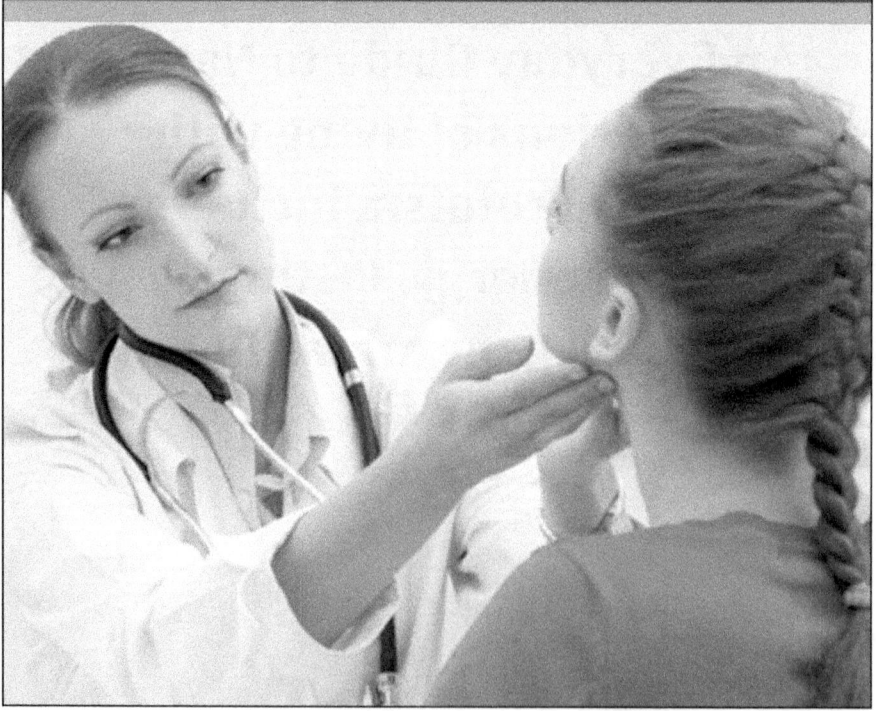

Table of Contents

Introduction

I want to thank you and congratulate you for purchasing the book, "The Hypothyroidism Handbook: An Everyday Guide to Natural solutions of living with Hypothyroidism including increased energy, lasting weight loss and general well-being".

This book contains proven steps and strategies on how to treat Hypothyroidism naturally. Hypothyroidism is known as the condition where in one has an abnormally low production of thyroid hormones. Lacks of thyroid hormones affect the body in many ways, such as:

- An enlarged heart

- Having a hard time losing weight which leads to too much weight gain

- Worsening heart failure

- Accumulation of fluid in the lungs which can lead to many respiratory diseases

With the help of this book, you will get to know the signs and symptoms of Hypothyroidism, its causes, and the various natural ways that you can combat the disease. If you want to live a long and healthy life without Hypothyroidism, you have to start reading this book now.

Thanks again for purchasing this book, I hope you enjoy it!

Chapter 1: Causes, Signs and Symptoms of Hypothyroidism

Before you get to know what could be done to fight off the disease, you should first get to know what causes it in the first place. Listed below are the most common causes of Hypothyroidism:

- **Pregnancy.** When women are pregnant or in that span of time just after giving birth, they tend to produce antibodies courtesy of their thyroid glands and that's why thyroid hormone production is lessened. The rise of blood pressure while pregnant may cause a miscarriage to happen or may affect the fetus.

- **Autoimmune Diseases**. Those who suffer from autoimmune diseases such as Hashimoto's Thyroditis are more likely to develop Hypothyroidism as their immune system is not working properly to protect them.

- **Radiation Therapy**. If you are already suffering from cancers of the neck and head that require radiation to be treated, you may also get to suffer from Hypothyroidism in the future.

- **Thyroid Surgery**. Of course, surgeries involving the thyroid can be big causes of Hypothyroidism because it halts or diminishes Thyroid Production.

- **Medication**. There are certain types of medicine that causes Hypothyroidism, especially those that are used to treat Psychiatric diseases such as Lithium. It would be best for you to ask your doctor about the certain effects of the medicines that you are taking to your body.

- **Pituitary Disorder.** Sometimes, the Pituitary gland fails to produce the enough number of Thyroid Stimulating Hormones or TSH because there are benign tumors in the Pituitary Gland. These then cause Hypothyroidism to happen.

- **Congenital Diseases.** Some babies are born with defective thyroid glands or no thyroid glands at all. It may be a cause of problems during pregnancy or because their parents also have Hypothyroidism.

- **Iodine Deficiency.** You know why they say that you have to eat foods that are rich in Iodine? Well, it's because Iodine Deficiency causes a lot of diseases such as Goiter and in this case, Hypothyroidism.

Common Symptoms of Hypothyroidism:

Be aware and see if you are suffering from Hypothyroidism. If you are experiencing some of the symptoms listed below, you probably are.

- Dry skin
- Constipation
- An increased insensitivity to coldness
- Having a puffy face
- Unexplained weight gain

- Weak muscles

- Hoarseness

- Feeling over-fatigued or exhausted most of the time

- Swelling of the joints, pain and stiffness

- Irregular menstrual periods

- Heavy menstrual periods

- Tenderness and stiffness of the muscles

- Impaired memory

- An unusual thinning of the hair

- Depression

- Slow heart rate

- Heightened blood cholesterol level

In infants, you have to be wary of the following:

- Frequent choking

- Yellowing of the white part of the eyes and of the skin, as well. This condition is also called Jaundice and happens when an infant's liver cannot metabolize Bilirubin, a substance that causes red blood cells to be damaged.

- A puffy face

- A protruding and large tongue

- Sleeplessness

- Constipation

And as for children and teens:

- Late development of permanent teeth

- Poor mental development

- Delayed growth, which often results to a short stature

- Delayed puberty or onset of menstruation for teenage girls

Take note that once Hypothyroidism is not treated early, it may worsen and that's why as early as now, you have to make sure that you keep yourself safe from the worsening of this disease. Turn to the next chapter and get to learn about the various ways of combating Hypothyroidism.

Chapter 2: Go Gluten Free!

A Gluten-free diet is said to be the most effective, natural way of getting rid of Hypothyroidism. This is a kind of diet that excludes the Protein Gluten from one's daily meals. This is because Gluten is said to be the cause of certain diseases such as Celiac Disease and is also known to damage one's intestines and thyroid glands.

A lot of people find it hard to just leave their old eating habits behind and switch to a Gluten-free kind of life. There's also the thought that one may not get all the nutrients that one's body needs and that are essential to one's growth, such as Iron and Calcium, but Gluten Diet practitioners say that the diet really has done wonders for them and that it can easily help someone to get healthier and be able to fight many diseases such as Hypothyroidism.

Which foods are allowed in this diet?

- Fresh eggs
- Unprocessed seeds, nuts and beans
- Fruits and vegetables
- Dairy products
- Fresh poultry, fish and meat which are not battered, marinated or coated
- Grains such as Buckwheat, Arrowroot, Flax, Corn, Cornmeal, Amaranth, Rice, Millet, Quinoa, Soy, Sorghum, Teff and Tapioca

Which foods should you avoid?

- Wheat

- Rye

- Barley, which means that you should also avoid beer, malt vinegar and malt flavoring that are made from Barley

- Triticale, a mix of wheat and rye

- Durum Flour

- Kamut

- Semolina

- Bulgur

- Farina

- Graham Flour

- Spelt

Aside from these, you should also avoid the foods listed below unless they are labeled as "Gluten-free":

- Pasta

- French Fries

- Gravy

- Candies, cookies and crackers

- Cereals

- Bread

- Salad dressings

- Seasoned potato chips and tortilla chips

- Seasoned rice mixes

- Soy sauce and other sauces

- Vegetables with sauce

- Self-basting poultry

- Processed or canned food such as Luncheon Meat and Corned Beef

- Soup bases and soup

With the right amount of discipline and self-control, you surely will be able to adhere to the Gluten Diet and allow yourself to live a longer and happier life. In the next chapter, you will learn about more ways of letting go of Hypothyroidism by means of what you eat.

Chapter 3: Eat your way to being healthy

If you cannot let go of your old eating habits and switch to the Gluten Diet easily, don't worry because you would still be able to combat the disease. You just have to be aware of what you eat and learn how to eat only nutritious kinds of food.

But what foods can help you in getting rid of Hypothyroidism? And what should you avoid? Here's what you need to know.

Get rid or eliminate coffee, sugar and carbohydrates

Eat non-starchy foods and vegetables, instead so that your body would be cleansed well and would not rely on sugar to live. Too much Sugar may also cause Hypothyroidism and other diseases such as Diabetes. Your body treats Carbohydrates like sugar and that's why you have to lessen your intake.

Fat can be your friend

Fat is considered as the great balancer of hormonal pathways—which means that you need to have them in your life. After all, if you are going to exercise after consuming some fat, you would be able to burn them away and still be in the right state of your body and in the target weight that you want to be in. You could get healthy fats from avocados, fish, nut butters, nuts, flax, Olive Oil, Ghee, full fat cheese, cottage cheese, yogurt and products made out of coconut milk.

Add Protein in your System

While Gluten is not allowed when it comes to beating Hypothyroidism, other kinds of Proteins are actually recommended for you. Right kinds of protein can be found in whole and grass-fed eggs, fresh fish, grass-fed meats, quinoa, nuts, and nut butters, as well.

Glutathione

More than the number of beauty products filled with Glutathione that have sprouted in the market like mushrooms, Glutathione is actually a healthy anti-oxidant that can be produced by the body by consuming certain kinds of food products, such as: raw eggs, avocados, garlic, squash, spinach, peaches, asparagus, broccoli, and grapefruit. Glutathione helps in producing thyroid hormones and protecting and healing thyroid glands. However, you should also take note that you have to control yourself from eating too much of some of them because they contain Goitrogens, which may interfere with the way your thyroid works. Foods rich in Goitrogen that must be lessened from your diet include:

Kale

- Rutabaga
- Broccoli
- Cauliflower
- Brussels Sprouts
- Millet
- Spinach

- Turnips

- Watercress

- Strawberries

- Peaches

- Peanuts

- Soybeans

- Radish

Take everything in moderation. Don't worry though because you do not have to completely eliminate them from your diet. Once cooked, these food products lose goitrogens. You just have to be careful about eating them raw and in large amounts.

Iodine

As mentioned earlier, Iodine is very important in keeping the body healthy and making sure that you are able to combat Hypothyroidism. It is also great in the prevention of diseases like cretinism, goiter, and mental disabilities, and also aids in the lessening of fatigue, lethargy, weight gain and depression. Iodine is essential in the production of thyroid hormones and that's why you have to include it in your diet. Aside from Iodized salt, which has been proven to reduce the number of patients affected with Hypothyroidism in the United States, other food products that are rich in Iodine include: Dried Seaweed, cod fish, unpeeled baked potato, fish sticks, shrimp, milk, canned tuna with oil, boiled egg, cooked navy beans and cooked turkey breast, as well.

Get rid of Inflammatory Foods

Inflammatory foods, or those that cause inflammation inside the body are a big no-no when it comes to fighting Hypothyroidism. People do not usually know which kinds of foods are considered inflammatory and that's why it is very important to check food labels in order for you to understand what it is that you will be eating. Inflammatory foods include:

- **Those with High Trans Fat**. Again, you have to check food labels for this. Trans fat is very inflammable and damages the cells that line your blood vessels which makes it very dangerous.

- **Cheeseburgers**. While they may be delicious and are great comfort foods, research has it that high amount of animal fat causes inflammation. Aside from that, cheeseburgers also cause tissue and gland damage—which might lead to Hypothyroidism instead of getting rid of it.

- **Sugar**. The body cannot break down each and every bit of sugar that you intake and that's why it is essential that you lessen the amount of sugar in your diet.

- **White bread.** This instantly breaks down to sugar as it is full of carbohydrates and as mentioned earlier, you do not need a lot of carbohydrates if you are trying to take care of yourself and trying to get rid of hypothyroidism. White bread makes the body more inflammable and that's not what you'd want to happen.

- **Alcohol**. Aside from the fact that beer is usually made from Barley, too much alcohol makes it easier for bacteria to make their way through your system and damage different tissues and organs. Alcohol also leads to inflammation—you've probably noticed this by the burning sensation you feel while drinking alcohol and just dismissed it as nothing, when in fact, it already damages your system.

- **Omega 6 Fatty Acids**. The difference of these from the healthy Omega 3 Fatty Acids is that they do not do the body good. Omega-6 rich foods include walnuts, vegetable oils and heavy seeds.

- **MSG**. You probably already know that MSG is bad for you and that's why you should cut back on junk foods. MSG can cause a lot of inflammation and may also cause diseases, especially thyroid and kidney related ones and that's why you should cut back on it.

- **Too much milk**. Again, you have to take everything in moderation because too much of anything is never a good thing. Don't drink too much milk especially if you are lactose-intolerant because you will not be able to digest it well.

Detoxify

Going on Detox is not just for those who are trying to get a great figure or are trying to diet just to look good. Detoxification is important for your body and mind to be rejuvenated and refreshed once again. There are so many juice cleanses available right now that you can choose from, or you can choose to make your own if that's more your thing. A combination of Chlorella, Turmeric, Cilantro and

Milk Thistle is said to be the best kind of juice cleanse mix that you can take in order to detoxify. You can also juice your choice of fruits and vegetables—what matters is that you drink them for them to work.

Keep these things in mind the next time you go grocery shopping or the next time you eat at a brand new restaurant. Your health should always be your top priority.

Chapter 4: Vitamins, Minerals, and Nutrients

Aside from eating the right kind of food, it is also very important for you to take the right kind of supplements and get the best nutrients for you to be able to fight Hypothyroidism well. Here are what you should intake, some foods included, and what you should avoid in order to be able to take care of your thyroid glands better and in order for your body to produce more thyroid hormones:

Stay away from BPA

BPA or Bisphenol A is commonly found in plastic bottles— the kind where you drink juices or teas or even water from. BPA damages your endocrine system and therefore, have bad effects on your thyroid. So, the next time you get thirsty, make it a point to drink only from glass or stainless steel cans. Also, look for the "BPA Free" sign from those plastic bottles to ensure that they are safe to use and drink from.

A Daptogen Supplements

A Daptogen Supplements are known to lower cortisol levels which in turn makes it easy for your thyroid glands to produce more thyroid hormones for you. You need A Daptogen to get rid of Adrenal Fatigue which is also one of the causes of Hypothyroidism. Tulasi, an herb cultivated for medicinal purposes which is also known as Holy Basil, and Ashwagandha or Winter Cherry are great sources of A Daptogen. As these herbs are more commonly found in India than in other parts of the world, taking supplements made out of them would be better than scouring the world to take hold of the herbs yourself.

A need for Selenium

Selenium, although not a very popular mineral, is actually important because it plays a key role in making metabolism faster. Once your metabolism is fast, it means that your body will be able to digest what you have been eating. This way, you're being able to combat Hypothyroidism. Aside from that, it is also known to battle other diseases such as Lung Cancer, Crohn's Disease and Prostate Cancer, as well.

Great sources of Selenium include: Grains, Poultry, Beef, Nuts, Brazil Nuts, Tuna, Herring, Red Snapper and Cod. Whole foods are also good sources of Selenium as the mineral gets dissolved once processing takes place.

Vitamin D

A walk in the sun before 10 am would be good to give your body the amount of Vitamin D that it needs to combat certain kinds of Cancer and Hypothyroidism, as well. Vitamin D3 supplements are also good to give you the Vitamin D that you lack in your system as lack of Vitamin D causes your glands not to produce thyroid hormones that are essential for you.

Iron

Iron is not only good for those who are suffering from Anemia, but is also good for your thyroid glands to produce more thyroid hormones that will help you become strong and will help you say goodbye to Hypothyroidism for good. Aside from taking Iron supplements, you may also eat foods that are rich in Iron, such as egg yolks, red meat, raisins, prunes, spinach, collards, beans, chick peas, lentils, soybeans, artichokes, liver, chicken giblets and turkey, as well. Take Iron along with Vitamin C and you surely will be able to combat the disease even better as Vitamin C is good against inflammation.

Probiotics

Probiotics are more commonly known as good bacteria. Your body needs these as they are the ones who get to fight bad bacteria from taking over your body. Good sources of Probiotics include:

- **Yogurt.** Yogurt is considered as the best source of Probiotics and is also considered as the best substitute for ice cream. Lactobacillus Shirota Strain-filled yogurt products are what you should go for. Aside from being good against Hypothyroidism, yogurt is also good for lessening gas, diarrhea and other kinds of digestive problems.

- **Kefir.** Kefir is a probiotic-filled drink that is said to have originated from Caucasus Mountains of Eurasia. It's almost the same as yogurt but is bubbly, creamy and thick and is good in battling yeast infections.

- **Milk with Probiotics.** There are some milk products that are made with probiotics. You'll know that they are if they are greenish in color and are creamier than your usual kind of milk. It is also commonly known as sweet acidophilus milk. Buttermilk is also known to be rich in probiotics so you can try that, as well.

- **Miso Soup.** Miso is quite popular in Japan and other parts of Asia as a soup made with fish and mustard plus the vegetable bok choi. A bowl of Miso soup contains at least 160 bacteria strains which are about the proper amount that you need each day. It is also low in calories and carbohydrates which make it perfect for someone who is trying to get rid of Hypothyroidism.

- **Sauerkraut**. These days, Sauerkraut is mainly used for sausage dishes and that's why you would not have a hard time trying to find it. Go for unpasteurized Sauerkraut because pasteurization is known to kill good bacteria.

- **Soft Cheese.** Gouda and other kinds of fermented cheese are able to survive in your system for a long time. This means that you will be safe from bad bacteria that damages cells and glands and so you will be able to eliminate the sources of Hypothyroidism.

- **Sourdough Bread.** Sourdough bread is popular for being great in making digestion and metabolism faster. It is also full of Lactobacilli, which are great examples of good bacteria.

- **Sour Pickles**. Pickles are also a good source of probiotics. Go for those that are naturally fermented or those that do not use vinegar in the fermentation process. These pickles also gave metabolic and digestive properties that are truly good for you.

- **Tempeh**. Tempeh is a popular kind of Indonesian Patty that is rich in natural antibiotics that fight bacteria and is also very high in protein. You would not have a hard time liking Tempeh because it is deliciously nutty and smoky and may also taste like a mushroom. You can also marinate Tempeh and add it to other dishes and recipes.

- **Or, you can just try taking Probiotic Supplements.** They are available in liquid, tablet or capsule form and will give you the right amount of Probiotics that you need.

Chapter 5: Thyroid Stimulating Exercises

Contrary to popular belief, there are actually some exercises that patients who suffer from Hypothyroidism can do. Just because you are suffering from Hypothyroidism does not mean that you can no longer workout or use your body for physical activities. Thinking this way would just worsen your disease.

Walking Daily

You'd be surprised to know how much walking contributes to your well-being. If you need to go somewhere and it's not far away from home, why not try walking instead of taking a can or riding other forms of public transport? Aside from the fact that you will be able to save some money, walking is simple and will also help you appreciate the beauty of your surroundings even better. Walking for around 20 to 40 minutes per day is already good to combat Hypothyroidism—it helps you lose weight and makes your metabolism faster. It also lets your thyroid glands work at an optimal rate.

Jogging

You don't need to do it professionally. Do it early in the morning or at night, upon coming home. You can do it in your own backyard if you want or use your village or the nearby park to jog. What's important is that you do it once or twice a week so that you'd get to burn all the extra fats that you have accumulated and so that your body will feel refreshed.

Circuit Training

Circuit Training is also proven to help reduce the risk of Hypothyroidism. Circuit Training also helps lower insulin levels, which in turn protects you against Diabetes. Some examples of these exercises include push-ups, lunges, curl-ups, bench presses, and sit ups for a couple of repetitions. If you do not like to go to the gym, then you can also do the exercises at the comforts of your own home. Rest a bit to catch your breath then do them again. You can devote at least 10 to 20 minutes of your day to Circuit Training and you will be alright.

Get to know your Acupressure Points

Devoting a bit of your time to massage or relax different Acupressure Points in your body would do wonders for your system when it comes to battling Hypothyroidism. You can do these for at least 2 to 5 times daily for them to work better. Some examples include:

- **Neck-Press.** Sit down and close your eyes and interlace your hands behind your neck, or on your nape. Bow your head down a bit and just relax. This way, you will be able to stretch your neck muscles. Then, bring your elbows together in front of you and compress the sides of your neck using your hands. Raise your head as you stretch gently and inhale and exhale as you relax. Repeat the exercise for at least 2 minutes.

- **K 27.** K 27 is known as both sides of your sternum. Just take long, deep breaths and turn your head from side to side. Allow yourself to feel how your neck region relaxes and just go and breathe deeply as you hold the K27 spots. Tilt your head up as you inhale, and down as you exhale and visualize the things that you want to have or the things you want to do someday. This is a good way of meditating, as well so not only do you help your body, you also get to clear your mind of its worries.

- **Temples.** Use your index and middle finger to massage your temples. Sit down, relax and massage both temples in circular motions. These will easily help you ease the pain that you are feeling and would also help you relax.

Chapter 6: Other Reminders

Aside from what was discussed in earlier chapters, here are some of the other things that you should keep in mind for you to be able to battle your disease.

Eliminate Stress

Stress causes you to feel bad about yourself, does not put your mind at ease, and also is one of the reasons why you get to suffer from some diseases such as Hypothyroidism because it causes your adrenal and thyroid glands to be exhausted. In order to eliminate stress, you should:

- **Try Meditation**. Go to a quiet place, think of a mantra, repeat it over and over again, and then make sure that you get to understand that it is true. For example, say "I can do this" or "I can get rid of this disease", and believe in it for it to be true. The power of positive thinking would really do you wonders so do not underestimate it.

- **Get an ample amount of sleep**. Sleeping for 6 to 8 hours each night, even if you are already an adult, is essential to help you become healthy and in top shape. If you get the right amount of sleep, you'd feel better about yourself and about the day that you are going to embark on. Getting the right amount of sleep equals happiness, so why would you deprive yourself of sleep?

- **Write your feelings down.** Creating a blog or writing on a journal always helps to make you feel better about yourself because you will be able to put your feelings out and let go of whatever it is that's bothering you. This way, you will be able to understand yourself better and get a clear mind when it comes to knowing that you will be able to battle the disease and let go of it—just as long as you believe that you can.

- **Do what you love.** It's much like a cliché, but doing what you love can do you wonders. When you know that you are doing things that people say you cannot do, or that are deemed as stupid, even if they are not, would surely make you feel better about yourself and would help lessen the stress in your life.

Drink lots of water

Another fact of life that most people take for granted is the fact that water is important to good health. It is also a given fact that drinking water is essential for those who have thyroid problems or thyroid related diseases. Aside from the traditional 8 glasses a day, you'd have to drink another glass for each pound that you want to lose.

Drink Green Tea

Research has it that aside from being able to cleanse your system, Green Tea is also good in making you more adept in exercising and in helping you feel better about yourself while exercising. And, it also calms you down which makes you feel less stressed and more motivated.

Remove Silver Fillings

If you've gotten treatment or Pasta for your teeth, you may have gotten silver fillings without being aware of it. These are also called Amalgam Fillings and may have high amounts of mercury which are dangerous to the body. It would be good to ask your dentist about what's in your Pasta before getting one, and if you already have one, then look for a dentist that offers Amalgam-free types of Pasta so that you will be safer. Amalgam also disrupts thyroid production and that's why you have to get rid of it.

And, Try Heat Therapy

Going to the sauna, taking a hot shower, or relaxing in a hot spring is great not only because they are able to help you relax and feel calmer, they are also able to eliminate stored toxins. It's important to get rid of the body's stored toxins as these only blocks the production of thyroid hormones which then causes Hypothyroidism.

Conclusion

Thank you again for purchasing this book!

I hope this book was able to help you to understand what Hypothyroidism is all about, how you will know that you have the disease and what to do to get rid of it.

The next step is to not only read and keep this book, but to actually try what is written in here. If you want to let go of your disease, then you should believe that you can and you should do whatever you can to let go of it and not let it take over your life. With the help of this book, you certainly can do it.

Finally, if you enjoyed this book, please take the time to share your thoughts and post a review on Amazon. We do our best to reach out to readers and provide the best value we can. Your positive review will help us achieve that. It'd be greatly appreciated!

Thank you and good luck!

Check Out My Other Books

Below you'll find some of my other popular books that are popular on Amazon and Kindle as well. Simply click on the links below to check them out. Alternatively, you can visit my author page on Amazon to see other work done by me.

Coconut Oil for Easy Weight Loss: A Step by Step Guide for Using Virgin Coconut Oil for Quick and Easy Weight Loss

http://www.amazon.com/Coconut-Oil-Easy-Weight-Loss-ebook/dp/B00JG8H8DE

Superfoods that Kickstart Your Weight Loss Learn How to Use 30 Superfoods to Boost Weight Loss, Immunity and to Live a Healthier Lifestyle

http://www.amazon.com/Superfoods-that-Kickstart-Your-Weight-ebook/dp/B00JNAPM9M

Carrier Oils for Beginners: Discover the Characteristics and Beauty and Health Benefits of Carrier Oils For mixing Aromatherapy Essential Oils

http://www.amazon.com/Carrier-Oils-Beginners-Characteristics-Aromatherapy-ebook/dp/B00K88GI2S

Natural Homemade Cleaning Recipes For Beginners: Essential Oil Recipes For Household Cleaning, Laundry & Toxic Free Living

http://www.amazon.com/Natural-Homemade-Cleaning-Recipes-Beginners-ebook/dp/B00K87UBQI

The Best Secrets of Natural Remedies: The Ultimate Guide to Natural Remedies to Prevent and Cure Illnesses, Cold and Flu for Your Family

http://www.amazon.com/Best-Secrets-Natural-Remedies-Illnesses-ebook/dp/B00JNDCOCM

The Hypothyroidism Handbook:An Everyday Guide to Natural Solutions of living with Hypothyroidism including increased energy, lasting weight loss, and general well-being

http://www.amazon.com/Hypothyroidism-Handbook-Solutions-including-increased-ebook/dp/B00JNIGIV0

The Hyperthyroidism Handbook: An Everyday Guide to Natural Solutions of Living with Hyperthyroidism including Weight Gain, Increased Energy and General Well-being

http://www.amazon.com/Hyperthyroidism-Handbook-Solutions-including-Hypothyroidism-ebook/dp/B00JOHU5SM

Essential Oils & Weight Loss for Beginners: Ultimate Guide to Losing Weight, Increasing Energy, Balancing Metabolism & Appetite Using Essential Oils & Aromatherapy

http://www.amazon.com/Essential-Oils-Weight-Loss-Beginners-ebook/dp/B00JOFOWP6

Top Essential Oil Recipes: A Recipe Guide Of Natural, Non-Toxic Aromatherapy & Essential Oils for Healing Common Ailments, Beauty, Stress & Anxiety

http://www.amazon.com/Top-Essential-Oil-Recipes-Aromatherapy-ebook/dp/B00JY434E2

Soap Making For Beginners: A Guide to Making Natural Homemade Soaps from Scratch, Includes Recipes and Step by Step Processes for Making Soaps

http://www.amazon.com/Soap-Making-Beginners-Homemade-Processes-ebook/dp/B00JYKH75I

Body Butters For Beginners: Proven Secrets To Making All Natural Body Butters For Rejuvenating And Hydrating Your Skin

http://www.amazon.com/Body-Butters-Beginners-Rejuvenating-Hydrating-ebook/dp/B00K6LVV6A

Apple Cider Vinegar For Beginners: Proven Secrets Using Apple Cider Vinegar For Health, Weight Loss, and Skin Care

http://www.amazon.com/Apple-Cider-Vinegar-Beginners-Aromatherapy-ebook/dp/B00K6YY6HI

Homemade Body Scrubs & Masks For Beginners: 50 Proven All Natural, Easy Recipes For Body & Facial Masks To Exfoliate Nourish, & Care For Your Skin

http://www.amazon.com/Homemade-Body-Scrubs-Masks-Beginners-ebook/dp/B00K79D4SY

Essential Oils Box Set #1: Essential Oils & Weight Loss For Beginners (Ultimate Guide to Losing Weight, Increasing Energy, Balancing Metabolism & Appetite Using Essential Oils & Aromatherapy) + Top Essential Oil Recipes (A Recipe Guide of Natural, Non-Toxic Aromatherapy & Essential Oils for Healing Common Ailments, Beauty, Stress & Anxiety) http://www.amazon.com/ESSENTIAL-OILS-BOX-SET-Aromatherapy-ebook/dp/B00K7Q8HRK

Essential Oils Box Set #2: Essential Oils & Weight Loss For Beginners (Ultimate Guide to Losing Weight, Increasing Energy, Balancing Metabolism & Appetite Using Essential Oils & Aromatherapy) + Top Essential Oil Recipes (A Recipe Guide of Natural, Non-Toxic Aromatherapy & Essential Oils for Healing Common Ailments, Beauty, Stress & Anxiety)

http://www.amazon.com/ESSENTIAL-OILS-BOX-SET-Aromatherapy-ebook/dp/B00K7Q8HRK

Box Set#3: Coconut Oil for Easy Weight Loss(A Step by Step Guide for Using Virgin Coconut Oil for Quick and Easy Weight Loss) + Apple Cider Vinegar(Proven Secrets Using Apple Cider Vinegar for Health, Weight Loss, and Skin Care)

http://www.amazon.com/Box-Set-Beginners-Aromatherapy-Essential-ebook/dp/B00K9TEGUW

Box Set #4: Body butters For Beginners(Proven Secrets To Making All Natural Body Butters For Rejuvenating And Hydrating Your Skin) & Top Essential Oil Recipes: A Recipe Guide Of Natural, Non-Toxic Aromatherapy & Essential Oils for Healing Common Ailments, Beauty, Stress & Anxiety

http://www.amazon.com/Box-Set-Butters-Beginners-Essential-ebook/dp/B00KA02F4Y

Box Set #5: Soap Making For Beginners(A Guide to Making Natural Homemade Soaps from Scratch, Includes Recipes and Step by Step Processes for Making Soaps) + Homemade Body Scrubs & Masks For Beginners(50 Proven All Natural,

Easy Recipes For Body Scrub & Facial Masks To Efoliate, Nourish, & Care For Your Skin)

http://www.amazon.com/Box-Set-Beginners-Homemade-Recipes-ebook/dp/B00K9U3I2I

Box Set #6: Body Butters for Beginners (Proven Secrets To Making All Natural Body Butters For Rejuvenating And Hydrating Your Skin) +Homemade Body Scrubs & Masks For Beginners(50 Proven All Natural, Easy Recipes For Body Scrub & Facial Masks To Exfoliate, Nourish, & Care For Your Skin)

http://www.amazon.com/Box-Set-Beginners-Exfoliating-Moisturizing-ebook/dp/B00K9U3Y4O

Box Set #7: TOP ESSENTIAL OILS(A Recipe Guide Of Natural, Non-Toxic Aromatherapy & Essential Oils For Healing, Common Ailments, Beauty, Stress & Anxiety) & THE BEST SECRETS OF NATURAL REMEDIES(The Ultimate Guide to Natural Remedies to Prevent and Cure Illnesses, Cold and Flu for Your Family)

http://www.amazon.com/BOX-SET-Essential-Recipes-Remedies-ebook/dp/B00K9WPMQG

Box Set #8: NATURAL HOMEMADE CLEANING RECIPES FOR BEGINNERS (Essential Oil Recipes for Household Cleaning, Laundry & Toxic Free Living) + TOP ESSENTIAL OILS(A Recipe Guide Of Natural, Non-Toxic Aromatherapy & Essential Oils For Healing, Common Ailments, Beauty, Stress & Anxiety)

http://www.amazon.com/BOX-SET-Beginners-Essential-Aromatherapy-ebook/dp/B00KAMNGBS

Box Set #9: Essential Oils & Weight Loss for Beginners (Ultimate Guide to Losing Weight, Increasing Energy, Balancing Metabolism & Appetite Using Essential Oils & Aromatherapy) + Carrier Oils for Beginners (Discover the Characteristics and Beauty and Health Benefits of Carrier Oils for Mixing Aromatherapy Essential Oils)

http://www.amazon.com/BOX-SET-Essential-Beginners-Aromatherapy-ebook/dp/B00KAODL6Q

BOX SET #10: THE HYPERTHYROIDISM HANDBOOK (An Everyday Guide to Natural Solutions of Living with Hyperthyroidism including Weight Gain, Increased Energy and General Well-being) + THE HYPOTHYROIDISM HANDBOOK (Everyday Guide to Natural Solutions of Living With Hypothyroidism Including Increased Energy, Lasting Weight Loss, and General Well-Being)

http://www.amazon.com/BOX-SET-10-Hyperthyroidism-Hypothyroidism-ebook/dp/B00KAKMSBY

BOX SET #11: CARRIER OILS FOR BEGINNERS (Discover the Characteristics and Beauty and Health Benefits of Carrier Oils for Mixing Aromatherapy Essential Oils) + Essential Oils & Aromatherapy for Beginners (Secrets to Beauty, Health and Weight Loss Using Proven Essential Oil and Aromatherapy Recipes

http://www.amazon.com/BOX-SET-Beginners-Essential-Aromatherapy-ebook/dp/B00KAONEQ8

BOX SET 12: ESSENTIAL OILS & WEIGHT LOSS FOR BEGINNERS: (Ultimate Guide to Losing Weight, Increasing Energy, Balancing Metabolism & Appetite Using Essential

Oils & Aromatherapy) + TOP ESSENTIAL OIL RECIPES (A Recipe Guide of Natural, Non-Toxic Aromatherapy & Essential Oils for Healing Common Ailments, Beauty, Stress & Anxiety) + CARRIER OILS FOR BEGINNERS (Discover the Characteristics & Beauty & Health Benefits of Carrier Oils for Mixing Aromatherapy Essential Oils) + ESSENTIAL OILS & AROMATHERAPY FOR BEGINNERS (Secrets to Beauty & weight Loss Using Proven Essential Oil & Aromatherapy Recipes) + NATURAL HOMEMADE CLEANING RECIPES FOR BEGINNERS (Essential Oil Recipes for Household Cleaning, Laundry & Toxic Free Living)

http://www.amazon.com/BOX-SET-12-Essential-Aromatherapy-ebook/dp/B00KCBCHE4

BOX SET #13: SUPERFOODS THAT KICKSTART YOUR WEIGHT LOSS (Learn How to Use 30 Superfoods to Boost Weight Loss, Immunity and to Live a Healthier Lifestyle) + ESSENTIAL OILS & AROMATHERAPY FOR BEGINNERS (Secrets to Beauty, Health and Weight Loss Using Proven Essential Oil and Aromatherapy Recipes) + BODY BUTTERS FOR BEGINNERS (Proven Secrets To Making All Natural Body Butters For Rejuvenating And Hydrating Your Skin) + SOAP MAKING FOR BEGINNERS (A Guide to Making Natural Homemade Soaps from Scratch, Includes Recipes and Step by Step Processes for Making Soaps) + HOMEMADE BODY SCRUBS FOR BEGINNERS (50 Proven All Natural, Easy Recipes For Body Scrub & Facial Masks To Exfoliate, Nourish, & Care For Your Skin)

http://www.amazon.com/BOX-SET-Superfoods-Kickstart-Aromatherapy-ebook/dp/B00KC8G6DK/

BOX SET 14: Essential Oils & Weight Loss for Beginners (Ultimate Guide to Losing Weight, Increasing Energy, Balancing Metabolism & Appetite Using Essential Oils & Aromatherapy) + Apple Cider Vinegar for Beginners (Proven Secrets Using Apple Cider Vinegar for Health, Weight Loss, and Skin Care) + Body Butters For Beginners (Proven Secrets To Making All Natural Body Butters For Rejuvenating And Hydrating Your Skin)
+ Homemade Body Scrubs & Masks for Beginners (50 Proven All Natural, Easy Recipes for Body Scrub & Facial Masks to Exfoliate, Nourish, & Care for Your Skin) + Coconut Oil for Easy Weight Loss (A Step by Step Guide for Using Virgin Coconut Oil for Quick and Easy Weight Loss)

http://www.amazon.com/BOX-SET-Essential-Beginners-Aromatherapy-ebook/dp/B00KEDO68U

www.ingramcontent.com/pod-product-compliance
Lightning Source LLC
Chambersburg PA
CBHW051239170526
45165CB00004B/1502